2024 12 LEAD EKG INTERPRETATION BASICS

Your ultimate knowledge-based guide to deciphering the heart's electrical language with confidence and precision

Gary Robin

Table Of Contents

How to Use This Guide

Welcome to "2024 12 Lead EKG Basics", your comprehensive companion on the journey to mastering EKG interpretation. This guide is designed to be user-friendly, engaging, and practical, ensuring that you not only learn but also enjoy the process. Here's how to make the most of this book and transform your EKG interpretation skills.

Start with the Basics

Before diving into complex arrhythmias and advanced interpretations, it's essential to build a solid foundation. The initial chapters of this book cover the fundamentals of EKGs, including understanding the machine, the basic waveforms, and the anatomy of a 12-lead EKG. By grasping these core concepts, you'll set yourself up for success in the more advanced sections.

Follow the Structured Approach

Each chapter is meticulously structured to build on the previous one. Start from the beginning and work your way through the book sequentially. This step-by-step approach ensures a gradual increase in complexity, allowing you to assimilate information without feeling overwhelmed. Take your time with each section, revisiting concepts as needed to reinforce your understanding.

Engage with Real-World Examples

Throughout the book, you'll find numerous real-world case studies and practice EKGs. These examples are designed to bridge the gap between theory and practice, providing you with hands-on experience in interpreting EKGs. Approach each case study as if you were in a clinical setting—analyze the EKG, apply the systematic interpretation method, and compare your findings with the detailed explanations provided.

Practice, Practice, Practice

Mastery of EKG interpretation comes with practice. The book includes a plethora of practice EKGs with detailed answers. Use these practice strips to test your knowledge and improve your skills. Try to interpret each EKG on your own before checking the explanations. This active practice will solidify your learning and boost your confidence.

Reflect and Review

At the end of each chapter, take a moment to reflect on what you've learned. Summarize the key points in your own words and review any sections that were challenging. Use the review questions and summaries provided to test your understanding. Regular reflection and review are crucial for long-term retention and mastery.

Connect the Dots

EKG interpretation is not just about reading lines on a strip; it's about understanding the heart's story. As you progress through the book, continuously connect the dots between the EKG patterns and the underlying cardiac physiology. Understanding the "why" behind each pattern will make you a more proficient and insightful interpreter.

Stay Curious and Engaged

Learning should be an enjoyable journey, not a chore. Approach each chapter with curiosity and enthusiasm. Engage with the content actively—ask questions, seek additional resources if needed, and apply your knowledge in clinical scenarios. The more engaged you are, the more rewarding the learning experience will be.

Utilize Additional Resources

While this book is a comprehensive guide, the world of EKG interpretation is vast. Don't hesitate to explore additional resources such as online courses, interactive EKG databases, and clinical practice. The combination of this guide and other learning tools will provide a well-rounded and robust education.

Seek Feedback and Collaborate

If possible, discuss your interpretations and findings with peers, mentors, or colleagues. Collaborative learning can provide new insights and perspectives, enhancing your understanding. Feedback from more experienced practitioners can also be invaluable in refining your skills.

Embrace Continuous Learning

The field of cardiology and EKG interpretation is always evolving. Stay updated with the latest guidelines, research, and advancements. View this book as the beginning of your journey, not the end. Embrace lifelong learning and continuously seek to improve your knowledge and skills.

Your Path to Mastery

"2024 12 Lead EKG Basics" is more than just a book; it's a gateway to mastering one of the most essential skills in healthcare. By following the structured approach, engaging actively with the content, and practicing diligently, you'll transform your ability to interpret EKGs accurately and confidently. This guide is your trusted companion, designed to support you every step of the way.

So, open the book, immerse yourself in the world of EKGs, and embark on this exciting journey to becoming an expert in EKG interpretation. Your patients and your practice will thank you for it. Happy reading, learning, and interpreting!

INTRODUCTION

Imagine a tool that can peer into the very essence of the heart, capturing its rhythms and revealing the secrets within its beats. Welcome to the world of 12-lead EKG interpretation—a fascinating journey into the heart's electrical activity. This book is your comprehensive guide to mastering the art of EKG interpretation, a skill that can save lives, improve patient care, and elevate your clinical expertise.

At the outset, let's talk about why this book exists and why it is essential. The purpose of this book is simple yet profound: to demystify the complexities of 12-lead EKG interpretation and provide you with a clear, systematic approach to understanding and interpreting EKGs. Whether you are a medical student just beginning your journey, a seasoned nurse seeking to enhance your skills, or a physician looking to refine your expertise, this book is designed for you. It aims to bridge the gap between theoretical knowledge and practical application, offering you the tools and confidence to accurately interpret EKGs.

The importance of EKG interpretation cannot be overstated. Electrocardiograms (EKGs) are indispensable in modern medicine, serving as a critical diagnostic tool in the assessment and management of numerous cardiac conditions. From the emergency room to the operating theater, from outpatient clinics to intensive care units, the ability to accurately read and interpret an EKG is a skill that transcends specialties and settings. A well-interpreted EKG can provide vital insights into the heart's function, reveal life-threatening conditions, guide treatment decisions, and monitor the effectiveness of interventions.

Let's take a moment to appreciate the wonder of the EKG. It's more than just a series of lines on a piece of paper or a screen; it's a real-time representation of the heart's electrical activity. Each wave and segment tells a story—a story of depolarization and repolarization, of electrical impulses traveling through the atria and ventricles, of the heart's intricate conduction system at work. Understanding this story requires both knowledge and intuition, a blend of science and art. This book is here to guide you through this journey, helping you develop the expertise needed to interpret EKGs with confidence and precision.

Now, who exactly is this book for? It's for anyone who wishes to master the skill of EKG interpretation, regardless of their level of experience or background. Medical students will find it an invaluable resource as they navigate their coursework and clinical rotations, providing a solid foundation that will serve them throughout their careers. Nurses, who often are the first to obtain and interpret EKGs, will benefit from the detailed explanations and practical tips, enhancing their ability to make quick, accurate assessments in fast-paced clinical environments. Paramedics and emergency medical technicians, who often encounter patients in critical conditions, will gain the skills needed to recognize and respond to cardiac emergencies swiftly and effectively.

For primary care physicians and specialists, this book offers a comprehensive review that reinforces their existing knowledge while introducing advanced concepts and nuances. Cardiologists, while already experts in the field, may find the systematic approach and case studies useful for teaching and refining their practice. Essentially, this book is for anyone involved in patient care who seeks to improve their EKG interpretation skills, whether you're a novice eager to learn or a veteran looking to stay sharp.

One of the most compelling aspects of EKG interpretation is its blend of simplicity and complexity. At its core, an EKG is a straightforward recording of the heart's electrical activity, but the interpretations that emerge from those squiggly lines can be profoundly intricate. This dichotomy is what makes EKGs so fascinating and, at times, challenging. By breaking down each component and building up your knowledge step by step, this book aims to make the complex more understandable and the simple more meaningful.

Consider the moment when you first glance at an EKG strip. To the untrained eye, it may seem like an indecipherable maze of peaks and troughs. But with knowledge and practice, each waveform begins to make sense. The P wave indicates atrial depolarization, the QRS complex represents ventricular depolarization, and the T wave signifies ventricular repolarization. These waves and complexes, though basic in their description, hold the key to diagnosing a myriad of cardiac conditions.

Imagine the satisfaction of identifying a myocardial infarction in its early stages, recognizing the telltale signs of atrial fibrillation, or pinpointing a bundle branch block. These are not just academic exercises; they are real-world skills that can change the course of a patient's life. Each EKG you interpret is a piece of the puzzle, providing crucial information that can guide your clinical decisions.

The journey to mastering EKG interpretation is akin to learning a new language. Initially, the characters and symbols seem foreign, the rules and syntax unfamiliar. But with time and practice, you begin to understand and even think in this new language. You start to see patterns, recognize abnormalities, and anticipate clinical implications. This book is your guide through this learning process, offering clear explanations, practical examples, and plenty of practice opportunities.

In writing this book, the goal has always been to make it as engaging and accessible as possible. Medical texts can sometimes be dry and difficult to read, but understanding EKGs should be an exciting and rewarding experience. Therefore, the language used is clear and conversational, the examples are relevant and relatable, and the illustrations are designed to enhance understanding. Learning should be enjoyable, and every effort has been made to ensure that this book is not only informative but also fun to read.

To keep you engaged, real-life case studies are included, providing context and demonstrating the application of concepts in clinical practice. These cases will challenge you to apply what you've learned, think critically, and develop a systematic approach to interpretation. By the end of this book, you will not only understand the mechanics of EKG interpretation but also appreciate its clinical relevance and importance.

Moreover, this book recognizes that everyone learns differently. Some may prefer detailed explanations and theoretical background, while others benefit from hands-on practice and visual aids. With this in mind, the content is presented in a variety of formats—text, diagrams, tables, and practice strips—to cater to different learning styles. Whether you're a visual learner who benefits from diagrams and illustrations or someone who learns best through repetition and practice, you'll find resources that suit your needs.

In conclusion, this book is more than just a manual; it's a journey into the heart of EKG interpretation. It's an invitation to explore the fascinating world of cardiac rhythms, to understand the nuances of heartbeats, and to gain a skill that can make a significant impact in the field of healthcare. Whether you're at the beginning of your career or looking to refine your expertise, this book offers something for everyone.

The heart's story is waiting to be told, and with this book, you'll have the tools to tell it. So, turn the page, start your journey, and immerse yourself in the art and science of 12-lead EKG interpretation. Your patients' hearts are counting on you.

Basics of EKG

Understanding the EKG Machine

Imagine stepping into a hospital room and seeing a machine with wires and leads connected to a patient. This device is an EKG machine, and it's one of the most powerful tools in modern medicine. Understanding how this machine works is the first step in mastering EKG interpretation.

An EKG machine is designed to detect the electrical activity of the heart. The heart generates electrical impulses that regulate its rhythm and contraction. These impulses are what the EKG machine records. The machine consists of several components: electrodes, leads, a display, and sometimes a printer.

Electrodes are small, sticky patches that are placed on the patient's skin. These electrodes detect the electrical activity of the heart. In a 12-lead EKG, there are typically ten electrodes placed in specific positions on the patient's chest and limbs. Each electrode picks up electrical signals from the heart, which are then transmitted to the EKG machine.

The leads are essentially the different views of the heart's electrical activity that the machine records. While we use ten electrodes, the 12-lead EKG provides twelve different perspectives on the heart's activity. This comprehensive view helps in accurately diagnosing various cardiac conditions.

Once the electrodes are placed and connected to the EKG machine, it begins to record the heart's electrical activity. This activity is displayed on a screen or printed on graph paper. The result is a series of waveforms that represent different phases of the heart's electrical cycle.

How EKGs Work

To appreciate how EKGs work, let's delve into the basics of cardiac electrophysiology. The heart has its own electrical system, which generates impulses that trigger heartbeats. These impulses start in the sinoatrial (SA) node, often referred to as the heart's natural pacemaker. Located in the right atrium, the SA node generates electrical impulses that spread throughout the atria, causing them to contract and push blood into the ventricles.

From the atria, the electrical impulse travels to the atrioventricular (AV) node, which acts as a gatekeeper. The AV node slows down the impulse before it moves into the ventricles. This delay allows the ventricles time to fill with blood before they contract. The impulse then travels down the bundle of His, which splits into the right and left bundle branches, and finally into the Purkinje fibers. These fibers spread the impulse throughout the ventricles, causing them to contract and pump blood to the lungs and the rest of the body.

The EKG machine captures these electrical impulses and displays them as waveforms. Each part of the waveform corresponds to a specific part of the heart's electrical cycle. By analyzing these waveforms, healthcare providers can determine if the heart's electrical activity is normal or if there are any abnormalities that need attention.

Basic EKG Waveforms

The EKG waveform is a graphical representation of the heart's electrical activity. It's divided into several key components: the P wave, the QRS complex, and the T wave. Each of these components tells a unique part of the heart's electrical story.

P Wave

The P wave represents atrial depolarization. Depolarization is a fancy term for the electrical activation of the heart's muscle cells. When the SA node fires, it sends an electrical impulse through the atria, causing them to contract and push blood into the ventricles. This electrical activity is captured as the P wave on the EKG. A normal P wave is small and rounded, indicating that the atria are depolarizing properly. Abnormalities in the P wave can suggest issues like atrial enlargement or atrial arrhythmias.

QRS Complex

Following the P wave is the QRS complex, which represents ventricular depolarization. This is when the electrical impulse travels through the ventricles, causing them to contract and pump blood out to the lungs and the rest of the body. The QRS complex is typically much larger than the P wave because the ventricles are larger and have more muscle mass. The QRS complex consists of three parts: the Q wave, the R wave, and the S wave. A normal QRS complex is narrow and sharp, indicating that the ventricles are depolarizing quickly and efficiently. A wide or abnormal QRS complex can suggest problems like ventricular hypertrophy, bundle branch blocks, or ventricular arrhythmias.

T Wave

After the QRS complex comes the T wave, which represents ventricular repolarization. Repolarization is the process of the heart's muscle cells resetting their electrical state in preparation for the next heartbeat. The T wave is usually smooth and rounded. Abnormalities in the T wave can indicate issues like electrolyte imbalances, ischemia, or ventricular hypertrophy.

By understanding these basic waveforms, you can begin to interpret the EKG and identify whether the heart's electrical activity is normal or abnormal. Each waveform provides clues about different parts of the heart's electrical cycle, and together they create a comprehensive picture of cardiac function.

To make this even more engaging, think of the EKG as a musical score. Just as a conductor reads the music to lead an orchestra, healthcare providers read the EKG to understand the heart's rhythm and identify any discordant notes. Each waveform is like a note on the score, contributing to the overall harmony of the heart's function. A skilled interpreter can quickly recognize when something is out of tune and take steps to correct it.

As you continue your journey into the world of EKG interpretation, remember that practice makes perfect. The more you familiarize yourself with these waveforms and their meanings, the more proficient you'll become at reading and interpreting EKGs. This skill will not only enhance your clinical practice but also improve the care you provide to your patients.

In conclusion, understanding the EKG machine, how EKGs work, and the basic waveforms are the foundational steps in mastering EKG interpretation. With this knowledge, you're well on your way to becoming proficient in this essential clinical skill. So, let's move forward and dive deeper into the fascinating world of EKG interpretation, one beat at a time.

12-Lead EKG Fundamentals

What is a 12-Lead EKG?

Imagine you have a camera that can take pictures from different angles, providing a complete view of an object. In the world of cardiology, a 12-lead EKG (electrocardiogram) works much like this multi-angle camera, capturing the electrical activity of the heart from various perspectives. This comprehensive snapshot allows healthcare professionals to assess the heart's function in great detail, making it an invaluable tool in diagnosing and managing heart conditions.

At its core, a 12-lead EKG records the electrical impulses that trigger heartbeats. These impulses travel through the heart, causing it to contract and pump blood. By placing electrodes on specific locations on the body, we can detect these electrical signals and create a detailed picture of the heart's activity. The term "12-lead" refers to the 12 different views or "leads" that the EKG machine generates, each providing a unique perspective of the heart's electrical activity.

Each lead corresponds to a specific axis or plane of the heart, allowing us to see different parts of the heart's electrical conduction system. For instance, some leads give us a view of the heart's frontal plane, while others provide insights into the heart's horizontal plane. By combining these views, we can identify abnormalities in the heart's rhythm, detect areas of poor blood flow, and diagnose conditions like heart attacks, arrhythmias, and more.

The beauty of a 12-lead EKG lies in its simplicity and effectiveness. With just a few electrodes and some basic knowledge, you can gain a wealth of information about the heart's health. It's a non-invasive, quick, and highly informative diagnostic tool that has become a staple in modern medicine.

Placement of Electrodes

To capture accurate and reliable EKG readings, precise placement of electrodes is crucial. Think of these electrodes as the "eyes" of the EKG machine, each positioned to capture a different view of the heart. Here's how you correctly place the electrodes for a 12-lead EKG:

1. Limb Electrodes:
   - Right Arm (RA): Place an electrode on the inner surface of the right arm, just above the wrist.
   - Left Arm (LA): Place an electrode on the inner surface of the left arm, just above the wrist.
   - Right Leg (RL): Place an electrode on the inner surface of the right leg, just above the ankle. This electrode serves as a ground and does not produce a lead.

- Left Leg (LL): Place an electrode on the inner surface of the left leg, just above the ankle.

2. Precordial (Chest) Electrodes:
- V1: Place the electrode in the fourth intercostal space (between the fourth and fifth ribs) just to the right of the sternum (breastbone).
- V2: Place the electrode in the fourth intercostal space just to the left of the sternum.
- V3: Position the electrode halfway between the positions of V2 and V4.
- V4: Place the electrode in the fifth intercostal space at the midclavicular line (an imaginary line drawn straight down from the middle of the clavicle or collarbone).
- V5: Place the electrode at the same level as V4, but at the anterior axillary line (an imaginary line running down from the front of the armpit).

- V6: Position the electrode at the same level as V4 and V5, but at the midaxillary line (an imaginary line running down from the middle of the armpit).

Accurate placement is essential because even small deviations can lead to incorrect interpretations. By placing the electrodes correctly, we ensure that the EKG readings are accurate, reliable, and useful for diagnosing heart conditions.

Lead Configurations and Views

Once the electrodes are in place, the EKG machine generates 12 leads, each providing a different view of the heart's electrical activity. These leads can be grouped into three main categories: limb leads, augmented limb leads, and precordial (chest) leads.

1. Limb Leads:
   - Lead I: Measures the electrical potential between the right arm and the left arm. It

provides a view of the heart's lateral (side) surface.

- Lead II: Measures the electrical potential between the right arm and the left leg. It gives a view of the heart's inferior (bottom) surface and is often used for rhythm analysis.

- Lead III: Measures the electrical potential between the left arm and the left leg. It also provides a view of the heart's inferior surface.

2. Augmented Limb Leads:

- aVR (augmented Vector Right): This lead is oriented towards the right arm, giving a unique perspective of the heart's electrical activity. It typically shows the inverse of what is seen in Lead II.

- aVL (augmented Vector Left): Oriented towards the left arm, this lead provides another lateral view of the heart.

- aVF (augmented Vector Foot): Oriented towards the feet, this lead offers a clear view of the heart's inferior surface.

3. Precordial (Chest) Leads:

   - V1 and V2: These leads provide views of the right ventricle and the interventricular septum (the wall separating the left and right ventricles).

   - V3 and V4: These leads focus on the anterior (front) part of the left ventricle.

   - V5 and V6: These leads provide views of the lateral surface of the left ventricle.

Each lead offers a unique vantage point, allowing for a comprehensive assessment of the heart's electrical activity. For instance, if there's an issue in the heart's inferior surface, it will be most apparent in leads II, III, and aVF. If there's a problem in the anterior surface, it will be reflected in leads V3 and V4. This multi-angle approach ensures that no area of the heart is left unexamined, enabling precise diagnosis and effective treatment planning.

Learning to interpret these leads takes practice and understanding, but once mastered, it becomes an invaluable skill. Think of each lead as a piece of a puzzle. Individually, they provide important information, but together, they create a complete picture of the heart's health. By systematically analyzing each lead, you can identify patterns, detect abnormalities, and make informed clinical decisions.

In conclusion, the 12-lead EKG is a powerful tool that offers detailed insights into the heart's electrical activity. Understanding the basics of what a 12-lead EKG is, how to place the electrodes, and how to interpret the lead configurations and views are essential steps in mastering this skill. With practice and patience, you will become proficient in reading EKGs, enabling you to provide better care for your patients and make a significant impact in the field of healthcare. So, let's dive in, explore the intricacies of the 12-lead EKG, and unlock the secrets of the heart together.

Normal EKG Interpretation

Understanding Normal Values

Welcome to the fascinating world of EKG interpretation! Let's start by getting a grip on the normal values you'll encounter on an EKG. Think of these values as your guideposts, helping you navigate through the complex terrain of cardiac rhythms. When we talk about "normal" EKG values, we're referring to the standard measurements that represent a healthy heart's electrical activity.

The first thing to know is the heart rate. A normal heart rate ranges from 60 to 100 beats per minute (bpm). This rate is measured by counting the number of QRS complexes (the spiky parts of the EKG) that occur in one minute. If the heart rate is below 60 bpm, it's called bradycardia. If it's above 100 bpm, it's known as tachycardia.

Next, let's talk about the P wave. The P wave represents atrial depolarization, which is the electrical activity that causes the atria (the upper chambers of the heart) to contract. A normal P wave is smooth and rounded, and it should be no more than 2.5 millimeters tall and 0.12 seconds wide.

Following the P wave is the PR interval, the time between the start of the P wave and the start of the QRS complex. This interval represents the time it takes for the electrical impulse to travel from the atria to the ventricles (the lower chambers of the heart). A normal PR interval ranges from 0.12 to 0.20 seconds. If the PR interval is longer than 0.20 seconds, it may indicate a delay in the electrical conduction system.

The QRS complex, which follows the PR interval, represents ventricular depolarization. This is when the ventricles contract to pump blood out to the body and lungs. A normal QRS complex is sharp and narrow, lasting less than 0.12 seconds. A wider QRS complex can indicate an abnormality in the way the ventricles are depolarizing.

After the QRS complex, we see the ST segment and the T wave. The ST segment represents the time between ventricular depolarization and repolarization (when the heart muscle prepares for the next beat). The ST segment should be flat and at the same level as the baseline of the EKG. Elevation or depression of the ST segment can indicate issues like ischemia or infarction (lack of blood flow to the heart muscle).

The T wave follows the ST segment and represents ventricular repolarization. A normal T wave is slightly asymmetrical and upright in most leads. It should not be too tall or too flat. Abnormalities in the T wave can suggest various cardiac conditions, such as electrolyte imbalances or myocardial infarction.

Finally, the QT interval, which includes the QRS complex, ST segment, and T wave, represents the total time for ventricular depolarization and repolarization. A normal QT interval is less than 0.44 seconds in men and less than 0.46 seconds in women. Prolongation of the QT interval can increase the risk of dangerous arrhythmias.

Understanding these normal values is crucial because they serve as the foundation for identifying abnormalities. Think of them as the "normal" setting on a radio. If the settings are off, you know something needs adjustment.

Systematic Approach to Reading EKGs

Reading an EKG can feel like solving a puzzle. To make this process easier, it's helpful to follow a systematic approach. This method ensures that you don't miss any critical details and helps you interpret EKGs consistently and accurately.

1. Rate: Begin by determining the heart rate. Count the number of QRS complexes in a 6-second strip and multiply by 10 to get the beats per minute. Alternatively, if you have a full 10-second strip, you can count the QRS complexes and multiply by 6.

2. Rhythm: Assess the regularity of the rhythm. Look at the spacing between QRS complexes. Is it regular or irregular? A regular rhythm has consistent spacing, while an irregular rhythm varies. This can help you identify arrhythmias.

3. P Waves: Examine the P waves. Are they present before each QRS complex? Are they smooth and rounded? This helps you determine if the atria are depolarizing normally.

4. PR Interval: Measure the PR interval. Is it within the normal range (0.12-0.20 seconds)? This tells you if there is any delay in the conduction from the atria to the ventricles.

5. QRS Complex: Check the QRS duration. Is it less than 0.12 seconds? A narrow QRS complex suggests normal ventricular depolarization, while a wide QRS can indicate a conduction delay or ventricular origin of the beat.

6. ST Segment: Evaluate the ST segment for elevation or depression. This can indicate ischemia, infarction, or other conditions affecting the heart muscle.

7. T Waves: Look at the T waves. Are they upright and asymmetrical? Abnormal T waves can suggest various cardiac issues.

8. QT Interval: Measure the QT interval. Is it within the normal range? Prolongation can predispose the patient to arrhythmias.

9. Overall Interpretation: Finally, put all the pieces together. Consider the clinical context and look for patterns that suggest specific conditions. This holistic view helps you make an accurate diagnosis.

By following this systematic approach, you can methodically analyze each part of the EKG and build a complete picture of the heart's electrical activity. Practice this method consistently, and soon it will become second nature.

Identifying Normal Sinus Rhythm

Normal sinus rhythm (NSR) is the gold standard for a healthy heart rhythm. Identifying NSR involves checking for specific criteria that indicate the heart's electrical system is functioning correctly.

First, the heart rate should be between 60 and 100 bpm. This range is considered normal for a resting adult. If the rate falls outside this range, it may indicate an arrhythmia, bradycardia, or tachycardia.

Next, look for the presence of P waves before each QRS complex. In NSR, every beat should originate from the sinoatrial (SA) node, the heart's natural pacemaker, which generates the P wave. The P waves should be consistent in shape and size, indicating that each beat is coming from the same place.

The PR interval should be within the normal range of 0.12 to 0.20 seconds. This interval represents the time it takes for the electrical impulse to travel from the atria to the ventricles. A normal PR interval suggests that the conduction pathway is clear and functioning properly.

The QRS complex should be narrow, less than 0.12 seconds, indicating that the ventricles are depolarizing normally. In NSR, the QRS complexes are evenly spaced, showing regular rhythm.

The ST segment should be flat, without any elevation or depression. This indicates that there is no acute ischemia or infarction affecting the heart muscle.

The T wave should be upright and slightly asymmetrical. It should follow the QRS complex without any significant delay. This shows normal ventricular repolarization.

Finally, the QT interval should be within the normal range for the patient's sex. A normal QT interval indicates that the ventricles are repolarizing within a safe timeframe, reducing the risk of arrhythmias.

To summarize, normal sinus rhythm is characterized by a heart rate of 60-100 bpm, consistent P waves before each QRS complex, a normal PR interval, narrow QRS complexes, flat ST segments, upright T waves, and a normal QT interval. Identifying these features confirms that the heart's electrical system is functioning as it should, providing a reliable baseline against which you can compare any abnormalities.

By mastering the identification of normal sinus rhythm, you lay the groundwork for recognizing deviations and diagnosing various cardiac conditions. With practice and repetition, you'll become proficient in quickly spotting NSR and understanding when something is amiss. This foundational skill is essential for anyone involved in cardiac care and will serve you well throughout your medical career.

Common EKG Abnormalities

Atrial Abnormalities

When we look at an EKG, we're not just seeing random lines; we're reading a story that the heart is telling us. Atrial abnormalities are among the most common issues you'll encounter, and they can tell us a lot about what's going on in the upper chambers of the heart, known as the atria.

One of the most frequent atrial abnormalities is atrial fibrillation, often referred to as "A-fib." Imagine the atria as a well-coordinated dance troupe. In a healthy heart, the dance is smooth and synchronized, but in atrial fibrillation, it's like each dancer is doing their own thing, leading to a chaotic performance. On an EKG, this looks like a wavy, irregular baseline instead of the neat, consistent P waves you'd expect with a normal rhythm. The QRS complexes—the sharp spikes that represent ventricular contractions—still appear, but they're irregularly spaced, reflecting the erratic signals from the atria.

Another common atrial abnormality is atrial flutter. Think of it as the atria trying to dance too fast. Instead of a chaotic performance like in A-fib, atrial flutter shows a very rapid but somewhat regular rhythm. On the EKG, this often looks like a sawtooth pattern, called "flutter waves," particularly noticeable in leads II, III, and aVF. The ventricles, receiving rapid-fire signals from the atria, usually respond at a regular rate but often more slowly than the flutter rate.

Atrial enlargement, another key abnormality, can also be identified on an EKG. When the atria are under strain, perhaps due to high blood pressure or valvular heart disease, they can enlarge, just like a muscle that's being overworked. This enlargement can be spotted on the EKG in the P waves. In right atrial enlargement, the P wave is tall and peaked, especially in lead II. Left atrial enlargement, on the other hand, shows up as a broad, often notched P wave, reflecting the prolonged depolarization as the electrical signal moves through the larger atrial muscle.

Ventricular Abnormalities

Moving down to the ventricles, the powerhouses of the heart, we encounter a different set of abnormalities. These abnormalities can be more serious because the ventricles are responsible for pumping blood throughout the body.

One of the most severe ventricular abnormalities is ventricular tachycardia, or "V-tach." Picture the ventricles racing uncontrollably, contracting so quickly that they can't properly fill with blood between beats. On an EKG, V-tach appears as a series of wide, bizarre QRS complexes, often at a rate of over 100 beats per minute. It's a medical emergency because it can lead to ventricular fibrillation, a chaotic rhythm where the ventricles quiver uselessly instead of pumping blood. Ventricular fibrillation, or "V-fib," looks like a chaotic, irregular waveform on the EKG, with no recognizable P waves, QRS complexes, or T waves. It's life-threatening and requires immediate intervention, usually defibrillation.

Another ventricular issue is premature ventricular contractions (PVCs). These are extra beats that occur when the ventricles fire off early, outside the normal rhythm. On the EKG, PVCs are seen as wide, bizarre QRS complexes that appear earlier than expected. They're often followed by a pause as the heart resets itself. While occasional PVCs are common and often harmless, frequent PVCs can indicate underlying heart problems and should be evaluated.

Bundle branch blocks are also significant ventricular abnormalities. The heart has two main branches in its conduction system, the left and right bundle branches. If one of these branches is blocked, it delays the electrical signal reaching that side of the heart. This delay shows up on the EKG as a widened QRS complex. In a right bundle branch block (RBBB), the QRS complex looks like an "M" or "rabbit ears" in leads V1 and V2, while in a left bundle branch block (LBBB), the QRS complex is wide and notched in leads V5 and V6.

Heart Blocks

Heart blocks are another critical category of EKG abnormalities, affecting the heart's ability to transmit electrical signals from the atria to the ventricles. These blocks can range from mild to severe and can significantly impact the heart's function.

First-degree heart block is the mildest form, where the electrical signal is delayed but still reaches the ventricles. On the EKG, this is seen as a prolonged PR interval, longer than 0.2 seconds. While usually not serious, it can indicate underlying heart conditions that need monitoring.

Second-degree heart block comes in two types: Mobitz Type I (Wenckebach) and Mobitz Type II. In Mobitz Type I, the PR interval progressively lengthens until a beat is dropped (the QRS complex fails to appear). This often looks like a repeating cycle on the EKG. Mobitz Type II, on the other hand, is more concerning. Here, the PR interval is constant, but occasional QRS complexes are dropped without warning. This irregularity can lead to more severe heart issues and often requires a pacemaker.

Third-degree heart block, or complete heart block, is the most severe form. In this condition, the atrial signals are completely blocked from reaching the ventricles. The atria and ventricles beat independently of each other, with the atria often at a normal rate and the ventricles at a much slower rate. On the EKG, this appears as P waves and QRS complexes that bear no relationship to each other. It's a serious condition that usually requires a pacemaker to ensure the heart beats effectively.

Understanding these common EKG abnormalities is crucial for anyone involved in patient care. Each abnormality tells a unique story about what's happening in the heart, providing vital clues that guide diagnosis and treatment. By recognizing these patterns and understanding their implications, you can make informed decisions that significantly impact patient outcomes.

In this book, we'll delve deeper into each of these abnormalities, exploring their causes, clinical significance, and management strategies. With practice and persistence, you'll become proficient in identifying and interpreting these key EKG findings, enhancing your ability to provide high-quality care to your patients. So, let's continue this journey into the fascinating world of EKG interpretation, where each beat tells a story, and every waveform holds a clue.

Advanced EKG Interpretation

Identifying Ischemia and Infarction

The heart, a powerful muscle tirelessly pumping blood, relies on a constant supply of oxygen and nutrients delivered by the coronary arteries. When these arteries become narrowed or blocked, the heart muscle (myocardium) suffers from a lack of oxygen—a condition known as ischemia. Prolonged ischemia can lead to myocardial infarction (MI), commonly known as a heart attack. Recognizing the signs of ischemia and infarction on an EKG is crucial for timely intervention and treatment.

Imagine a scenario: you are in the emergency room, and a patient arrives complaining of chest pain. The first tool you reach for is the EKG. Understanding what to look for on this seemingly simple strip of paper can make a life-saving difference.

Ischemia

Ischemia is the early stage of oxygen deprivation in the heart muscle. On an EKG, ischemia typically presents as changes in the ST segment and T waves. The ST segment is the flat section of the EKG between the end of the S wave (part of the QRS complex) and the beginning of the T wave.

- ST Segment Depression: One of the hallmark signs of ischemia is ST segment depression. This means that the ST segment is lower than the baseline. It can appear as a horizontal, down-sloping, or up-sloping depression. A significant ST depression (more than 1 mm) is a red flag, indicating that part of the heart muscle isn't getting enough oxygen.

- T Wave Inversion: Another clue is the inversion of T waves, which means the T wave points downward instead of upward. This change can be subtle or pronounced, but it often accompanies ischemic conditions.

Infarction

When ischemia progresses and the heart muscle starts to die, we enter the territory of myocardial infarction (MI). The EKG changes associated with an MI are more dramatic and evolve through different stages:

- Hyperacute T Waves: In the very early stages of an MI, the T waves may become tall and peaked. This stage is fleeting and can be easily missed if the EKG is not done promptly.

- ST Segment Elevation: The most telling sign of an acute MI is ST segment elevation. Unlike ST depression, elevation means that the ST segment is higher than the baseline. This elevation represents injury to the heart muscle and is a medical emergency. The specific pattern and location of ST elevation can help determine which part of the heart is affected. For example, ST elevation in leads II, III, and aVF indicates an inferior MI, while elevations in leads V1-V4 suggest an anterior MI.

- Pathological Q Waves: As the infarction progresses, pathological Q waves may develop. These Q waves are deeper and wider than normal and signify that a part of the heart muscle has undergone irreversible damage. Once they appear, they typically remain on the EKG indefinitely, serving as a marker of a past MI.

- T Wave Inversion: After the acute phase, T wave inversion can reappear and persist for days, weeks, or even longer, reflecting ongoing changes in the heart muscle as it heals.

Bundle Branch Blocks

The heart's electrical system is like a well-choreographed dance, with impulses traveling down specific pathways to ensure the heart beats in a coordinated manner. These pathways include the right and left bundle branches. When one of these branches is blocked, the result is a bundle branch block (BBB), which disrupts the normal sequence of electrical activation.

Right Bundle Branch Block (RBBB)

In a right bundle branch block, the electrical impulse is delayed as it travels to the right ventricle. This delay results in a distinctive pattern on the EKG.

- QRS Duration: The QRS complex is wider than usual, typically greater than 120 milliseconds (three small squares on the EKG paper).

- RSR' Pattern: In leads V1 and V2, which look at the right side of the heart, you'll see a pattern that looks like rabbit ears or an "M" shape. This is due to the delayed depolarization of the right ventricle.

- Wide S Waves: In the lateral leads (I, aVL, V5, V6), you might notice wide, slurred S waves.

RBBB can be seen in healthy individuals but may also indicate underlying heart disease, especially if it appears suddenly.

Left Bundle Branch Block (LBBB)

Left bundle branch block involves a delay in the electrical impulse as it travels to the left ventricle, creating a different but equally distinctive pattern.

- QRS Duration: Like RBBB, the QRS complex in LBBB is also widened, exceeding 120 milliseconds.

- Notched R Waves: In leads that view the left side of the heart (I, aVL, V5, V6), you'll see broad, notched R waves, which may look like the top of a mountain.

- Absent Q Waves: The normal small Q waves in these leads are absent in LBBB.

- Deep S Waves: In the right precordial leads (V1, V2), deep, broad S waves are present.

LBBB is often associated with significant underlying heart disease, such as coronary artery disease or cardiomyopathy, and warrants further investigation.

Axis Deviation

The heart's electrical axis represents the general direction of the electrical impulse as it travels through the heart. Think of it as the compass direction of the heart's electrical activity. Axis deviation occurs when this direction shifts abnormally, either to the left or the right.

Determining the Axis

To determine the axis, we look at the QRS complexes in leads I and aVF:

- Normal Axis: If the QRS complexes in both leads I and aVF are positive (pointing upward), the axis is normal, generally between -30° and +90°.

- Left Axis Deviation (LAD): If the QRS complex in lead I is positive and in lead aVF is negative, the axis is deviated to the left, between -30° and -90°. LAD can indicate conditions like left ventricular hypertrophy, left anterior fascicular block, or a prior inferior MI.

- Right Axis Deviation (RAD): If the QRS complex in lead I is negative and in lead aVF is positive, the axis is deviated to the right, between +90° and +180°. RAD may be seen in conditions such as right ventricular hypertrophy, chronic lung disease, or left posterior fascicular block.

Clinical Relevance of Axis Deviation

Understanding axis deviation helps in diagnosing and understanding the underlying cardiac or systemic conditions affecting the heart. It provides a clue about the heart's structural and functional status, guiding further diagnostic and therapeutic steps.

Interpreting advanced EKGs involves not just recognizing patterns, but understanding the story behind those patterns. It's about connecting the dots between the electrical impulses we see on the EKG and the physiological events happening in the heart. By mastering the interpretation of ischemia, infarction, bundle branch blocks, and axis deviation, you gain a powerful tool in your clinical arsenal, one that can significantly impact patient care and outcomes. With practice, what may seem like a bewildering array of lines and waves transforms into a coherent, informative narrative of the heart's health and function.

Clinical Correlation

As we delve deeper into the fascinating world of EKG interpretation, it's essential to connect the dots between what we see on the EKG and what is happening in the patient's body. Clinical correlation is about understanding how specific EKG changes reflect various cardiac and systemic conditions. This chapter will explore EKG changes associated with three common and critical conditions: myocardial infarction, pericarditis, and pulmonary embolism. To make these concepts come alive, we'll also examine real-life case studies, giving you a practical understanding of how to apply this knowledge.

EKG Changes in Various Conditions

Myocardial Infarction (MI)

Myocardial infarction, commonly known as a heart attack, occurs when blood flow to a part of the heart muscle is blocked. This can lead to damage or death of the heart muscle if not treated promptly. EKG changes are crucial in diagnosing and managing MI. Here's what you need to look for:

1. ST-Elevation Myocardial Infarction (STEMI)

- ST Segment Elevation: One of the hallmark signs of a STEMI is the elevation of the ST segment. This elevation occurs because of the injury to the heart muscle. On the EKG, it appears as a noticeable upward deflection of the ST segment from the baseline.

- Reciprocal Changes: These are ST segment depressions in leads opposite to those showing elevation. They provide further confirmation of myocardial infarction.

- Q Waves: Pathological Q waves can develop hours to days after an infarct, indicating necrosis (death) of heart muscle tissue. These waves are wider and deeper than normal Q waves.

2. Non-ST-Elevation Myocardial Infarction (NSTEMI)

- ST Segment Depression: Unlike STEMI, NSTEMI often shows ST segment depression or T wave inversions. These changes reflect ischemia (reduced blood flow) rather than full-thickness injury.

- T Wave Inversions: These indicate ischemia and are common in NSTEMI. They may persist for weeks after the event.

Pericarditis

Pericarditis is inflammation of the pericardium, the thin sac-like membrane surrounding the heart. EKG changes in pericarditis are distinctive and can help differentiate it from other conditions like MI.

1. Diffuse ST Elevation: Unlike the localized ST elevation seen in STEMI, pericarditis typically causes diffuse (widespread) ST segment elevation across multiple leads.

   - Concave Upward ST Elevation: The ST segment elevation in pericarditis often has a concave (saddle-shaped) appearance, which is different from the convex (tombstone) appearance in STEMI.

   - PR Segment Depression: Another key feature is the depression of the PR segment, most evident in the lead II and other limb leads.

2. Stage Progression: Pericarditis evolves through stages, with initial ST elevation followed by normalization, then T wave

inversions, and eventually normalization of T waves.

Pulmonary Embolism (PE)

A pulmonary embolism is a blockage in one of the pulmonary arteries in the lungs, usually caused by blood clots that travel from the legs or other parts of the body (deep vein thrombosis). While EKG is not the primary diagnostic tool for PE, it can provide important clues.

1. Sinus Tachycardia: The most common finding in PE is sinus tachycardia, an increased heart rate.

   - S1Q3T3 Pattern: This classic but not universally present pattern involves a deep S wave in lead I, a Q wave in lead III, and an inverted T wave in lead III. It suggests right heart strain due to a large PE.

- Right Bundle Branch Block (RBBB): RBBB or incomplete RBBB can appear in PE, indicating increased pressure in the right ventricle.

- Right Axis Deviation: This deviation occurs due to right ventricular strain or hypertrophy.

Case Studies

To bring these concepts to life, let's explore some real-life scenarios.

Case Study 1: Myocardial Infarction

Patient Background:

John, a 55-year-old male, arrives at the emergency room complaining of severe chest pain radiating to his left arm and jaw. He is diaphoretic and short of breath.

Initial EKG Findings:

The EKG shows significant ST segment elevation in leads II, III, and aVF with reciprocal ST segment depression in leads I and aVL. Additionally, there are Q waves developing in the inferior leads.

Clinical Correlation:

These EKG changes are indicative of an inferior wall myocardial infarction. The presence of reciprocal changes and Q waves further confirms the diagnosis. John is immediately started on aspirin, nitroglycerin, and is prepared for urgent coronary angiography.

Outcome:

Coronary angiography reveals a complete occlusion of the right coronary artery. John undergoes successful percutaneous coronary intervention (PCI) with stent placement.

Follow-up EKG shows resolution of ST elevation and improved clinical condition.

Case Study 2: Pericarditis

Patient Background:

Maria, a 30-year-old female, presents with sharp chest pain that worsens when lying down and improves when sitting up. She reports a recent history of a viral upper respiratory infection.

Initial EKG Findings:

The EKG shows diffuse ST segment elevation in almost all leads, with the most pronounced in leads I, II, and V3-V6. The ST segments have a concave upward appearance. Additionally, there is PR segment depression in lead II.

Clinical Correlation:

These findings are classic for acute pericarditis. The diffuse nature of the ST elevation and the presence of PR segment depression, along with Maria's clinical history, support this diagnosis. Maria is treated with nonsteroidal anti-inflammatory drugs (NSAIDs) and colchicine for inflammation.

Outcome:

Over the next few days, Maria's symptoms improve significantly. A follow-up EKG shows resolution of ST elevation and normalization of the PR segment. She continues to recover without complications.

Case Study 3: Pulmonary Embolism

Patient Background:

Robert, a 45-year-old male with a history of deep vein thrombosis, presents with sudden onset of shortness of breath and chest pain. He has tachycardia and hypotension.

Initial EKG Findings:

The EKG shows sinus tachycardia with a heart rate of 120 beats per minute. There is an S1Q3T3 pattern: a deep S wave in lead I, a Q wave, and an inverted T wave in lead III. There is also evidence of right axis deviation.

Clinical Correlation:

The EKG findings suggest right heart strain consistent with a significant pulmonary embolism. The S1Q3T3 pattern, sinus tachycardia, and right axis deviation point towards this diagnosis. Robert is started on anticoagulation therapy and undergoes a CT pulmonary angiography, which confirms a large embolism in the right pulmonary artery.

Outcome:

Robert is treated with thrombolytic therapy due to the severity of his symptoms. He stabilizes over the next 24 hours, and subsequent EKGs show improvement in the strain pattern. He is discharged on long-term anticoagulation and referred for follow-up care.

Understanding the clinical correlation between EKG changes and various conditions is a critical aspect of mastering EKG interpretation. By recognizing specific patterns associated with myocardial infarction, pericarditis, and pulmonary embolism, you can make timely and accurate diagnoses, guiding appropriate management and improving patient outcomes. Through the lens of case studies, we've seen how these principles apply in real-world scenarios, reinforcing the importance of a systematic and informed approach to EKG interpretation. As you continue to practice and refine your skills, these insights will become second nature, empowering you to make a significant impact in the care of your patients.

Practical Tips and Tricks

Interpreting an EKG can seem daunting at first, but with practice and a few handy tips and tricks, you'll find it becomes much easier and even enjoyable. In this chapter, we'll explore common pitfalls that many beginners encounter and provide you with practical advice to help you interpret EKGs quickly and accurately.

Common Pitfalls in EKG Interpretation

When starting out with EKG interpretation, it's easy to make mistakes. Here are some common pitfalls and how to avoid them:

1. Not Using a Systematic Approach

One of the most common mistakes is not following a systematic approach. Skipping steps or interpreting findings in isolation can lead to errors. Always use a step-by-step method: rate, rhythm, axis, intervals, waveforms, and any abnormalities.

2. Ignoring Patient History and Clinical Context

EKG interpretation should never be done in a vacuum. Always consider the patient's history and clinical presentation. For example, what might look like a benign finding in a healthy young adult could be significant in an elderly patient with a history of heart disease.

3. Overlooking Calibration and Lead Placement Issues

Before interpreting an EKG, ensure that the machine calibration is correct and the leads are properly placed. Incorrect lead placement can result in misleading EKG tracings, leading to incorrect diagnoses.

4. Misidentifying Normal Variants as Pathological

It's essential to recognize that there are normal variants in EKG readings. For instance, early repolarization can look concerning but is a normal finding in young, healthy individuals. Understanding what constitutes a normal variant can prevent unnecessary alarm.

5. Misinterpreting Artifact as Abnormality

Electrical interference, muscle tremors, and patient movement can create artifacts that resemble pathological findings. Always check if the pattern is consistent across leads or if it matches known artifacts.

6. Failure to Recognize Subtle Changes

Subtle changes can be easily missed, especially when they involve only a few millimeters of deviation. Always compare with previous EKGs if available and be thorough in your analysis.

7. Over-Reliance on EKG Machines

Modern EKG machines often provide automated interpretations. While these can be helpful, they are not foolproof. Always verify the machine's interpretation with your own assessment.

By being aware of these common pitfalls, you can take proactive steps to avoid them, ensuring more accurate EKG interpretations.

Tips for Quick Interpretation

Interpreting an EKG quickly doesn't mean rushing through it; it means being efficient and effective. Here are some tips to help you speed up the process without compromising accuracy:

1. Develop a Routine

Having a consistent, systematic approach is key. Start by checking the calibration and lead placement. Then, analyze the rate, rhythm, axis, intervals, waveforms, and any abnormalities in the same order every time. This routine helps ensure nothing is overlooked.

2. Use Mnemonics

Mnemonics can be incredibly helpful for remembering the steps and components of EKG interpretation. One popular mnemonic is "Rate, Rhythm, PQRST":

- Rate: Calculate the heart rate.
- Rhythm: Determine if the rhythm is regular or irregular.
- P wave: Check for the presence and morphology of P waves.
- QRS complex: Analyze the QRS duration and morphology.

- ST segment and T wave: Look for any deviations or abnormalities.

3. Quickly Assess the Rate

Counting the number of R waves in a 6-second strip and multiplying by 10 gives you a quick estimate of the heart rate. Alternatively, for regular rhythms, use the "300, 150, 100, 75, 60, 50" rule by dividing 300 by the number of large squares between R waves.

4. Rhythm at a Glance

For rhythm assessment, look at the regularity of the R-R intervals. Regular intervals suggest a regular rhythm, while variable intervals suggest an irregular rhythm. Also, check if there is a P wave before every QRS complex to assess atrioventricular (AV) association.

5. Focus on Key Leads

Certain leads provide more information for specific conditions. For example:

- Lead II: Excellent for assessing atrial activity and rhythm.

- Leads V1 and V6: Helpful for evaluating ventricular activity and bundle branch blocks.

- Leads I, II, and aVF: Useful for determining the heart's electrical axis.

6. Spot Common Abnormalities

Familiarize yourself with common EKG patterns and abnormalities, such as:

- Atrial fibrillation: Irregularly irregular rhythm without distinct P waves.
- ST elevation: Indicative of myocardial infarction.

- T wave inversions: Can signify ischemia or other conditions.
- Wide QRS complex: May indicate a bundle branch block or ventricular rhythm.

7. Practice, Practice, Practice

The more EKGs you interpret, the more proficient you'll become. Practice with a variety of EKGs, from normal to highly abnormal, to build your skills and confidence.

8. Use Technology Wisely

There are many excellent apps and online resources that provide EKG practice strips, tutorials, and even interactive quizzes. These tools can supplement your learning and provide additional practice opportunities.

9. Stay Updated

EKG interpretation guidelines can evolve. Stay current by reading relevant medical literature, attending workshops, and participating in continuing education courses.

10. Seek Feedback

If you're in a learning environment, ask for feedback from experienced colleagues or mentors. Discussing your interpretations and learning from others can significantly enhance your skills.

As you continue to practice and apply these tips, you'll find that EKG interpretation becomes less daunting and more intuitive. Remember, becoming proficient takes time and patience, so keep practicing and learning.

In summary, interpreting EKGs accurately and efficiently is a skill that combines knowledge, practice, and a systematic approach. By avoiding common pitfalls and employing practical tips and tricks, you can develop the confidence and expertise needed to make critical clinical decisions based on EKG findings. Embrace the journey of mastering EKG interpretation, and you'll discover a fascinating world that enhances your understanding of the heart and improves patient care.

Practice EKGs

Sample EKGs for Practice

As you embark on the journey of mastering EKG interpretation, practice is essential. To truly understand and become proficient at reading EKGs, you need to see a variety of examples and learn how to interpret them. In this chapter, you will find a collection of sample EKGs that represent common scenarios you might encounter in clinical practice. Each example will be accompanied by a detailed explanation to guide you through the interpretation process. So, let's dive in and start decoding these fascinating heart rhythms.

Sample EKG 1: Normal Sinus Rhythm

Let's start with the basics—a normal sinus rhythm. Understanding what a normal EKG looks like is crucial before moving on to abnormal patterns.

![EKG Image - Normal Sinus Rhythm](https://www.example.com/normal-sinus-rhythm.png)

Interpretation Steps:

1. Rate: Count the number of QRS complexes in a 6-second strip and multiply by 10 to get the heart rate per minute. In this example, you see 8 QRS complexes, so the heart rate is 80 beats per minute (bpm).

2. Rhythm: Look for regularity. The R-R intervals are consistent, indicating a regular rhythm.

3. P Waves: Check if each P wave is followed by a QRS complex. Here, every P wave is followed by a QRS, and the P waves are upright and uniform.

4. PR Interval: Measure the distance from the start of the P wave to the start of the

QRS complex. It should be between 0.12 to 0.20 seconds. This example shows a PR interval of 0.16 seconds.

5. QRS Duration: Measure the width of the QRS complex. It should be less than 0.12 seconds. Here, the QRS duration is 0.08 seconds.

Conclusion: This EKG shows a normal sinus rhythm, which is what you should expect in a healthy individual.

Sample EKG 2: Sinus Bradycardia

Next, let's look at an example of sinus bradycardia, where the heart rate is slower than normal.

Interpretation Steps:

1. Rate: Count the QRS complexes. In this 6-second strip, there are 5 QRS complexes, indicating a heart rate of 50 bpm.

2. Rhythm: The R-R intervals are regular.

3. P Waves: Each P wave is followed by a QRS complex.

4. PR Interval: The PR interval is within normal limits, measured at 0.18 seconds.

5. QRS Duration: The QRS complex duration is 0.08 seconds.

Conclusion: This EKG demonstrates sinus bradycardia, a slower than normal heart rate but otherwise normal conduction.

Sample EKG 3: Atrial Fibrillation

Now, let's examine a more complex rhythm—atrial fibrillation.

Interpretation Steps:

1. Rate: The rate is variable in atrial fibrillation, but you can estimate an average. In this example, the heart rate is approximately 110 bpm.

2. Rhythm: The R-R intervals are irregular.

3. P Waves: There are no discernible P waves; instead, there are erratic, fibrillatory waves.

4. PR Interval: Not measurable due to the absence of consistent P waves.

5. QRS Duration: The QRS complexes are narrow, with a duration of 0.08 seconds.

Conclusion: This EKG shows atrial fibrillation, characterized by an irregular rhythm and absence of P waves.

Sample EKG 4: Ventricular Tachycardia

Let's move on to an example of a potentially life-threatening arrhythmia—ventricular tachycardia.

Interpretation Steps:

1. Rate: The heart rate is very rapid, around 180 bpm.

2. Rhythm: The rhythm is regular.

3. P Waves: P waves are typically not visible in ventricular tachycardia.

4. PR Interval: Not measurable.

5. QRS Duration: The QRS complexes are wide, exceeding 0.12 seconds, often around 0.16 seconds.

Conclusion: This EKG indicates ventricular tachycardia, a dangerous condition requiring immediate medical attention.

Detailed Explanations and Answers

Understanding the "why" behind each interpretation is critical for mastering EKG reading. Here, we will delve deeper into the detailed explanations for each sample EKG.

Normal Sinus Rhythm Explanation

A normal sinus rhythm is the gold standard for comparing other EKGs. It signifies that the heart's electrical activity is functioning correctly, starting from the sinoatrial (SA) node, which is the natural pacemaker. The P waves indicate atrial depolarization, the QRS complex shows ventricular depolarization, and the T wave represents ventricular repolarization.

Sinus Bradycardia Explanation

Sinus bradycardia is a slower than normal heart rate but follows the same electrical pathway as normal sinus rhythm. It can be seen in healthy individuals, especially athletes, and during sleep. However, it can also indicate issues like hypothyroidism, increased intracranial pressure, or the effects of certain medications.

Atrial Fibrillation Explanation

Atrial fibrillation is a common arrhythmia where the atria beat irregularly and often rapidly, leading to poor blood flow and increased risk of stroke. The absence of P waves and the presence of irregularly irregular R-R intervals are key identifiers. Treatment may involve rate control, rhythm control, and anticoagulation therapy to prevent thromboembolic events.

Ventricular Tachycardia Explanation

Ventricular tachycardia (VT) is a serious condition that can lead to ventricular fibrillation and sudden cardiac arrest. It originates from the ventricles, and the wide QRS complexes reflect abnormal conduction. VT can be caused by structural heart disease, electrolyte imbalances, or myocardial infarction. Immediate intervention, such as antiarrhythmic drugs, cardioversion, or defibrillation, may be necessary.

By practicing with these sample EKGs and understanding the detailed explanations, you will build the confidence and skill needed to interpret a wide range of EKGs accurately. Remember, each EKG you encounter is an opportunity to apply your knowledge and improve your interpretation skills. Keep practicing, stay curious, and soon the once-mysterious lines on the EKG paper will tell a clear and compelling story.

Conclusion

As we draw this journey to a close, it's time to reflect on the wealth of knowledge you've acquired and the skills you've honed throughout this book. The realm of 12-lead EKG interpretation is vast and intricate, yet profoundly rewarding. Each chapter has been a step toward mastering the art of reading the heart's electrical activity, a skill that is as critical as it is life-saving.

Remember when we first started, deciphering those initial, seemingly cryptic lines and waves? What once appeared as an indecipherable code now tells a clear and detailed story. You've learned to see beyond the surface of the EKG strip, delving into the heart's rhythm and beats to uncover the secrets within. This transformation, from novice to knowledgeable interpreter, is a testament to your dedication and curiosity.

Throughout this book, we've explored the fundamentals, from the basic components of an EKG to the intricacies of a 12-lead setup. We've demystified the normal sinus rhythm, the cornerstone of EKG interpretation, providing a solid foundation upon which all other interpretations are built. Understanding what is normal is crucial, as it allows you to recognize when something is amiss, a skill that is invaluable in clinical practice.

We ventured into the world of arrhythmias, learning to identify common and uncommon patterns that indicate various cardiac conditions. From the slow beats of sinus bradycardia to the chaotic waves of atrial fibrillation, you've gained the ability to recognize and understand the implications of these rhythms. More importantly, you've learned to respond to them, understanding the clinical significance and potential treatments.

The journey didn't stop there. We tackled more complex interpretations, including the identification of ischemia and infarction, conditions that require prompt and accurate diagnosis. The ability to recognize these patterns can make a critical difference in patient outcomes, highlighting the importance of your skills.

One of the most enriching parts of this journey has been the practical application of knowledge through case studies and practice EKGs. These real-world examples bridged the gap between theory and practice, allowing you to test and refine your skills in a safe, educational environment. Each case study was an opportunity to apply what you've learned, to think critically, and to develop a systematic approach to EKG interpretation.

But the journey of learning never truly ends. The heart, with its complexities and nuances, always has more to teach us.

Continue to practice, to read, and to seek out new experiences. Every EKG you interpret is another step toward mastery, another opportunity to improve your understanding and sharpen your skills.

This book has equipped you with a robust toolkit. You've learned to measure and analyze the rate, rhythm, and morphology of EKGs. You can now identify key features and abnormalities, understand their clinical implications, and make informed decisions based on your interpretations. These skills are not just academic; they are practical and essential, impacting the care you provide to your patients.

As you move forward, take with you the systematic approach that has been emphasized throughout this book. Always start with the basics—rate, rhythm, and intervals—before moving on to more complex analyses. This methodical approach ensures that no detail is overlooked, leading to accurate and thorough interpretations.

Your journey in EKG interpretation is also a journey of growth as a healthcare professional. The ability to read and interpret EKGs enhances your diagnostic capabilities, broadens your clinical acumen, and ultimately improves the quality of care you provide. It's a skill that brings you closer to your patients, allowing you to understand their hearts in the most literal sense.

In conclusion, mastering 12-lead EKG interpretation is both a challenge and a privilege. It's a skill that requires ongoing practice, a keen eye for detail, and a deep understanding of cardiac physiology. But it's also a skill that brings immense rewards, both professionally and personally. The knowledge you've gained empowers you to make critical decisions, to act swiftly in emergencies, and to provide comprehensive care to your patients.

As you close this book, take pride in what you've accomplished. You've embarked on a journey into the heart of medicine, one that will continue to unfold with every EKG you interpret. Keep learning, keep practicing, and let your passion for understanding the heart drive you forward. The heart's story is ever-evolving, and with the skills you've developed, you're now well-equipped to read and respond to it.

Thank you for allowing this book to be a part of your journey. Here's to your continued growth, to the lives you will impact, and to the heartbeats you will understand. The world of EKG interpretation is at your fingertips—embrace it with confidence and curiosity.

www.ingramcontent.com/pod-product-compliance
Lightning Source LLC
Chambersburg PA
CBHW071941210526
45479CB00002B/773